I am a KIDNEY DISEASE WARRIOR

20 Strengthening Sayings to Color

kathy WELLER

I Am A Kidney Disease Warrior: 20 Strengthening Sayings To Color ©2018 Kathy Weller

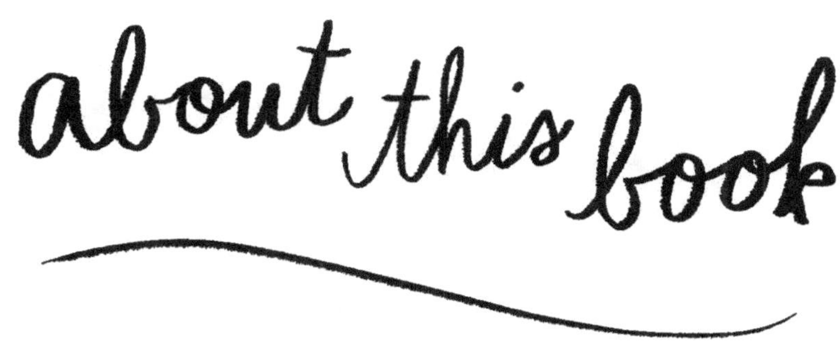

When my 91-year-old great aunt Eadie was diagnosed with kidney failure, we had to learn about the options that were available to her, and quickly. What we learned is that kidney disease and it's treatment options can be scary, nerve-wracking, and very difficult to manage. We discovered that management is very dependent on age and on the unique existing health factors of each individual.

Dialysis? Eadie wasn't a candidate for either type. But before we knew that, we learned all about it: The physical treatment aspects, what it demands of the person mentally, physically, emotionally, and in terms of the time commitment.

It hit me like a hurricane: Kidney disease requires a person's complete and total commitment, in EVERY facet of their life. If dialysis is a part of the treatment plan, super-powered mental strength and physical stamina, not to mention the aforementioned lifestyle change, are not negotiable. There is no sugar-coating it: Kidney disease should have the motto "For Warriors Only". Because that's the truth. THAT is what you are.

Eadie passed away a couple of months ago. While she was still here, she was my sounding board and consultant for the empowering phrases in this book. I know Eadie would love that this book now exists to help others to stay positive and in a good mindset to slay their diagnosis. Look: YOU are— basically— super-human. Don't doubt it. And, stay strong!! This book is for you. I'm with you all the way. So is Eadie... and so is this book, any time you need it.

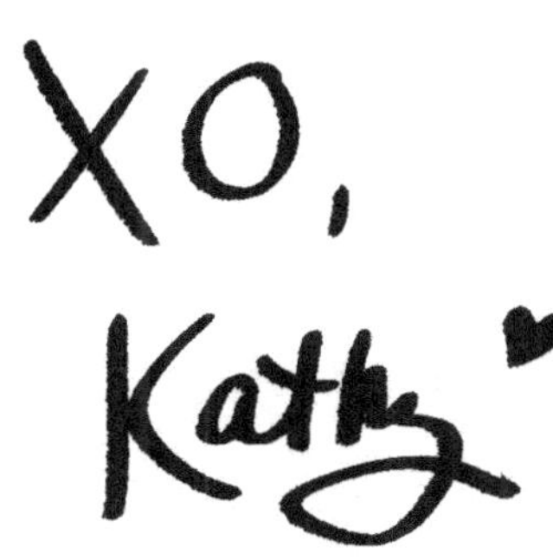

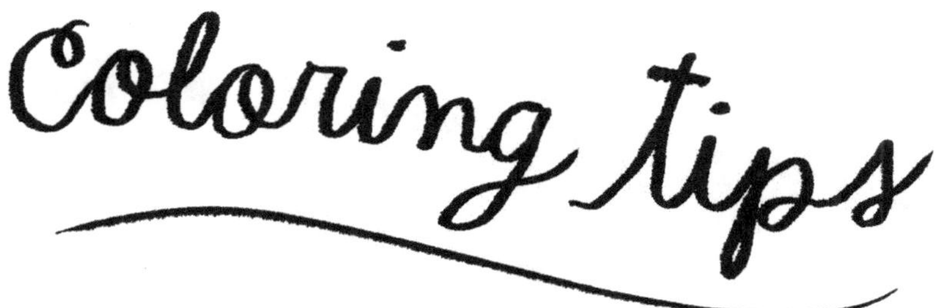

Coloring tips

 The paper in this book does well with dry media such as colored pencils, caran d'ache neocolor pastels, and other types of oil pastels and crayons.

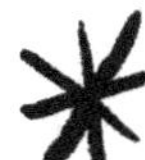 Markers of all types are fine, but please place a page or two of plain paper underneath the page being colored on to prevent any bleed-through.

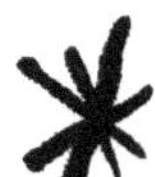 The images to color are printed on one side of the paper, with the other side left intentionally blank.

 Some of the illustrations feature darker, thicker black lines. They're there for variety, to emphasize parts of the design, and to give you flexibility for exploration with opaque drawing media, like gel pens and crayons!

 I made an effort to balance each coloring design with a little extra space in the book binding area. This was done to make it easier for you to cut the page out, if you wish to.

 Have fun!

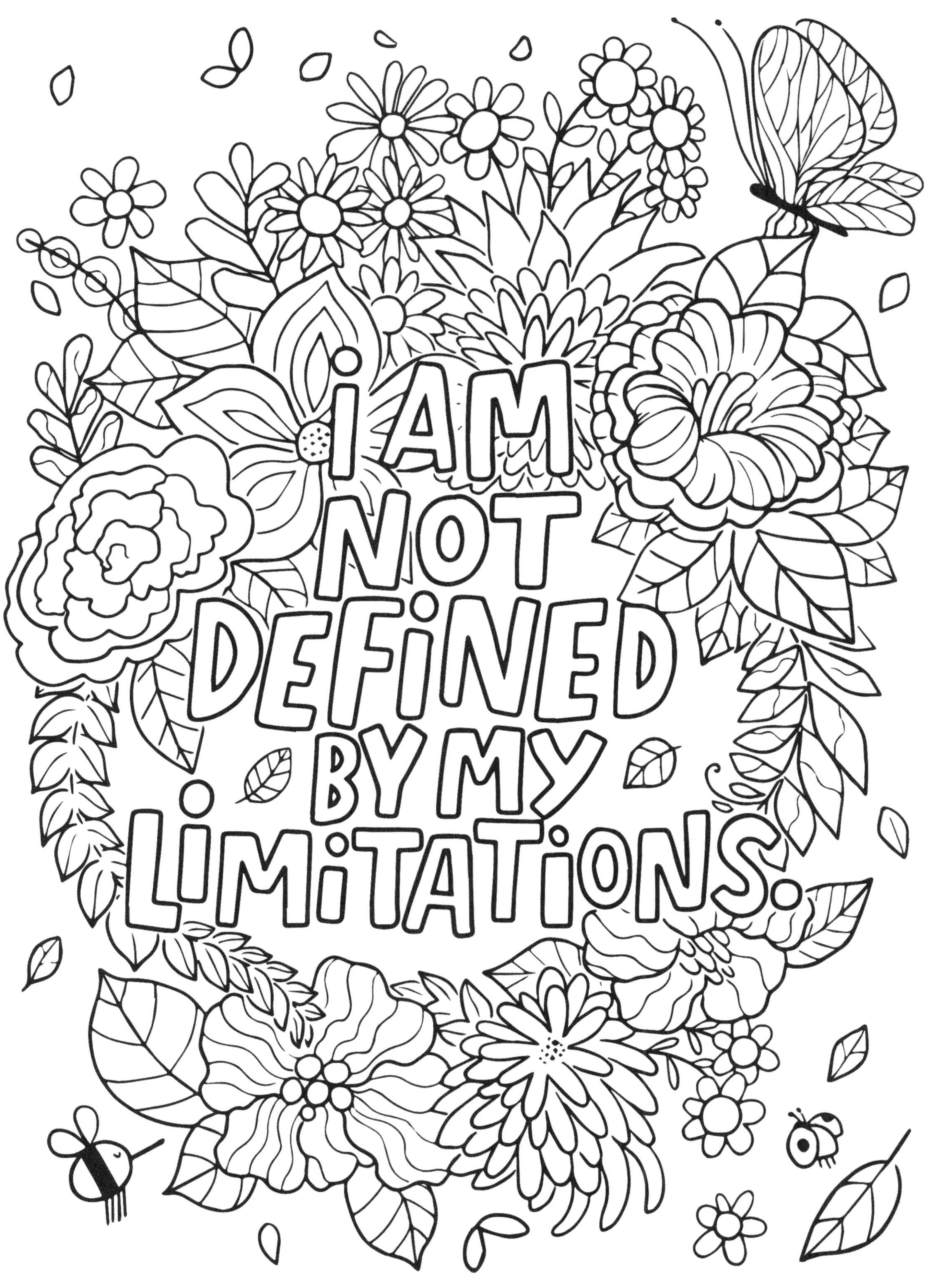

I AM
NOT
DEFINED
BY MY
LIMITATIONS.

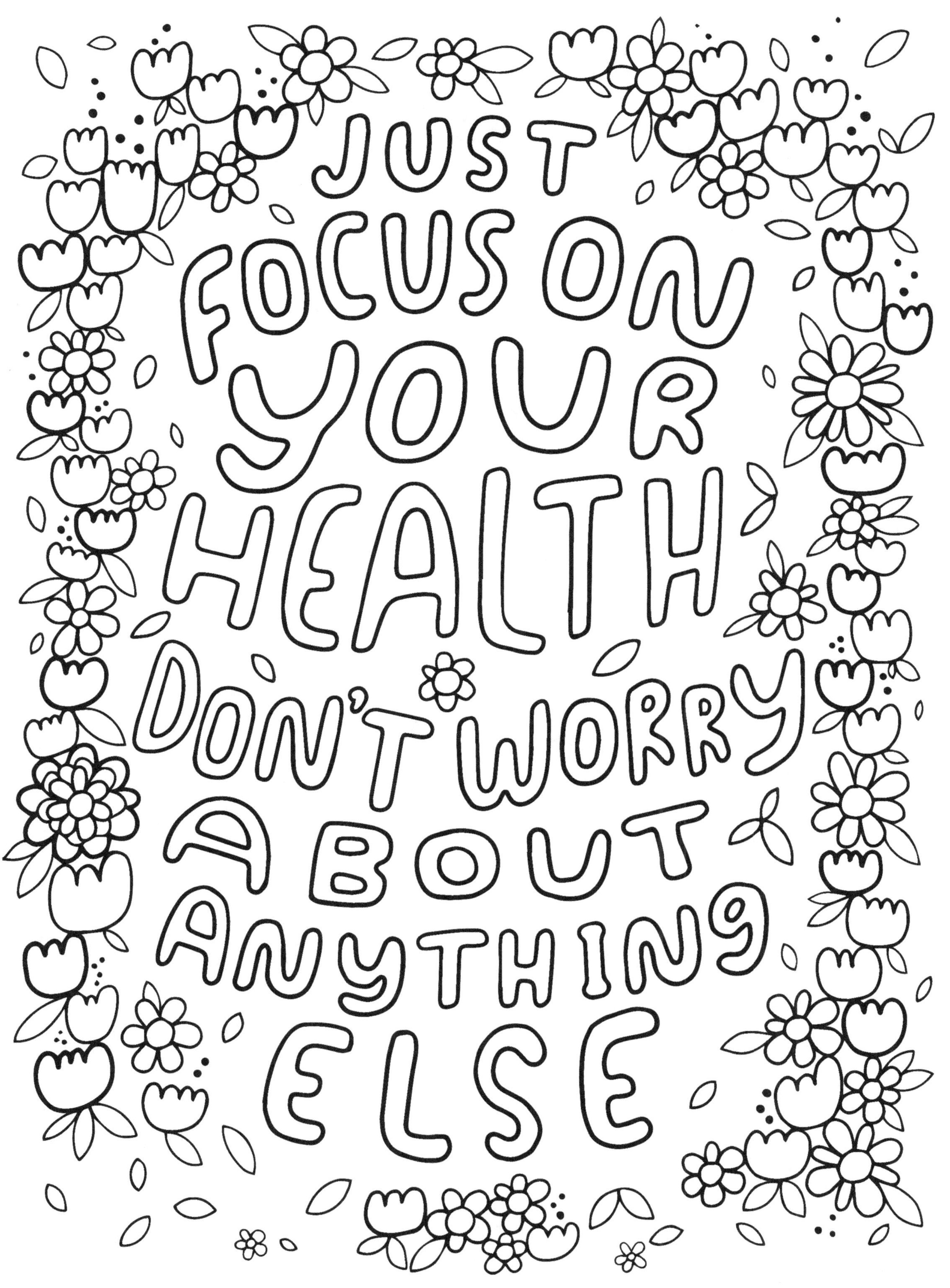

JUST
FOCUS ON
YOUR
HEALTH
DON'T WORRY
ABOUT
ANYTHING
ELSE

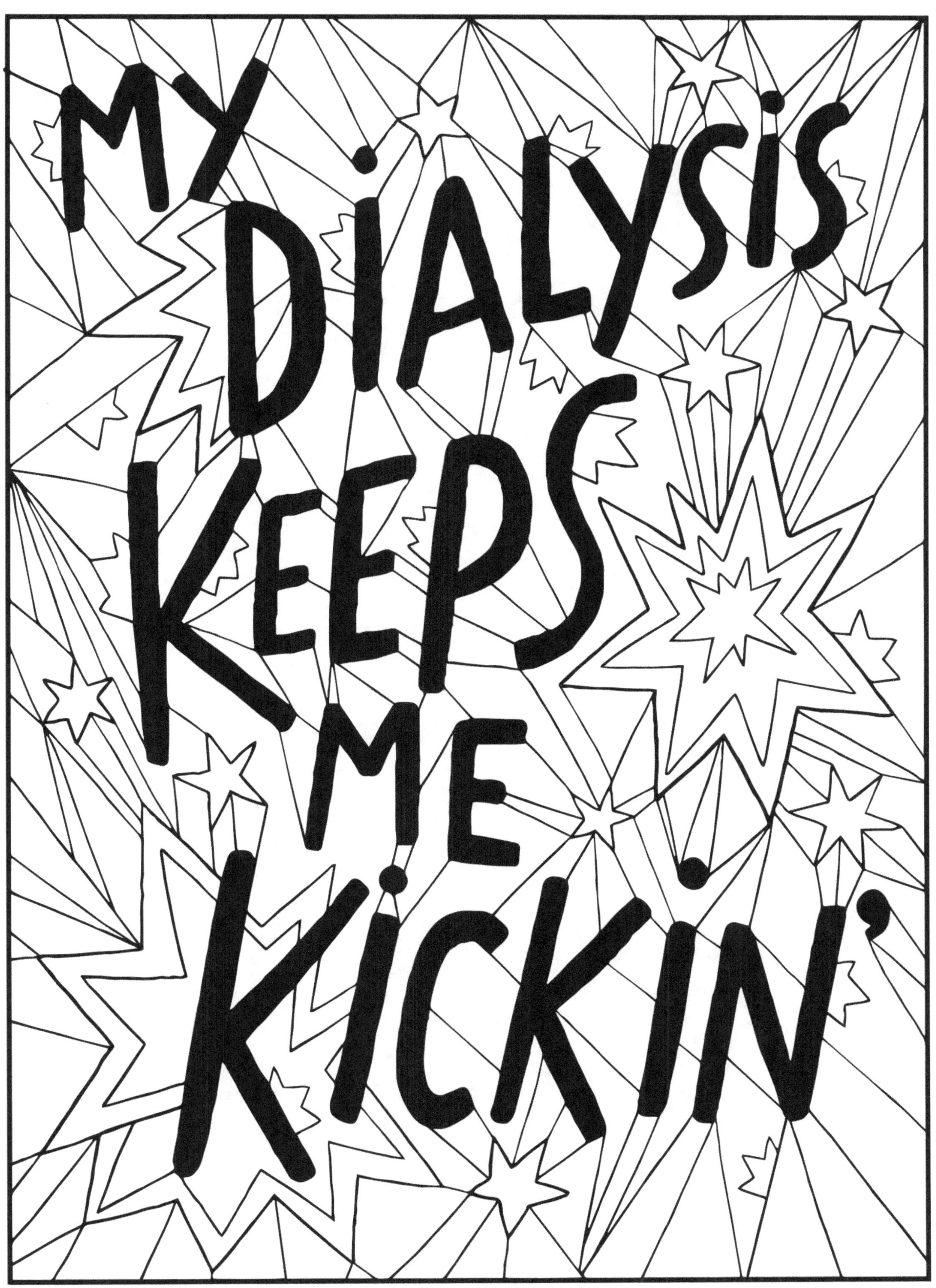

MY DIALYSIS KEEPS ME KICKIN'

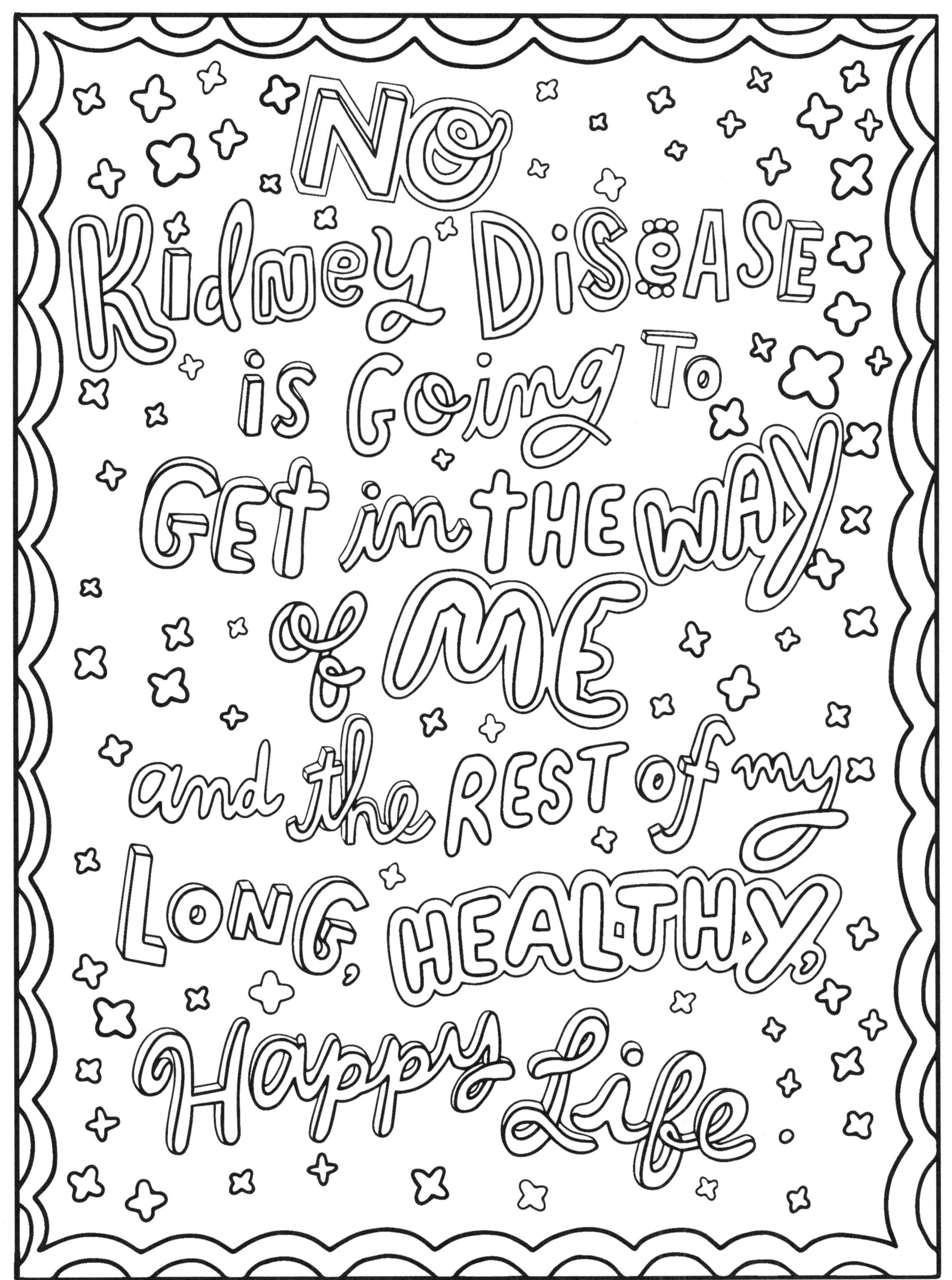

No
Kidney Disease
is Going To
Get in the Way
of Me
and the Rest of my
Long, Healthy,
Happy Life.

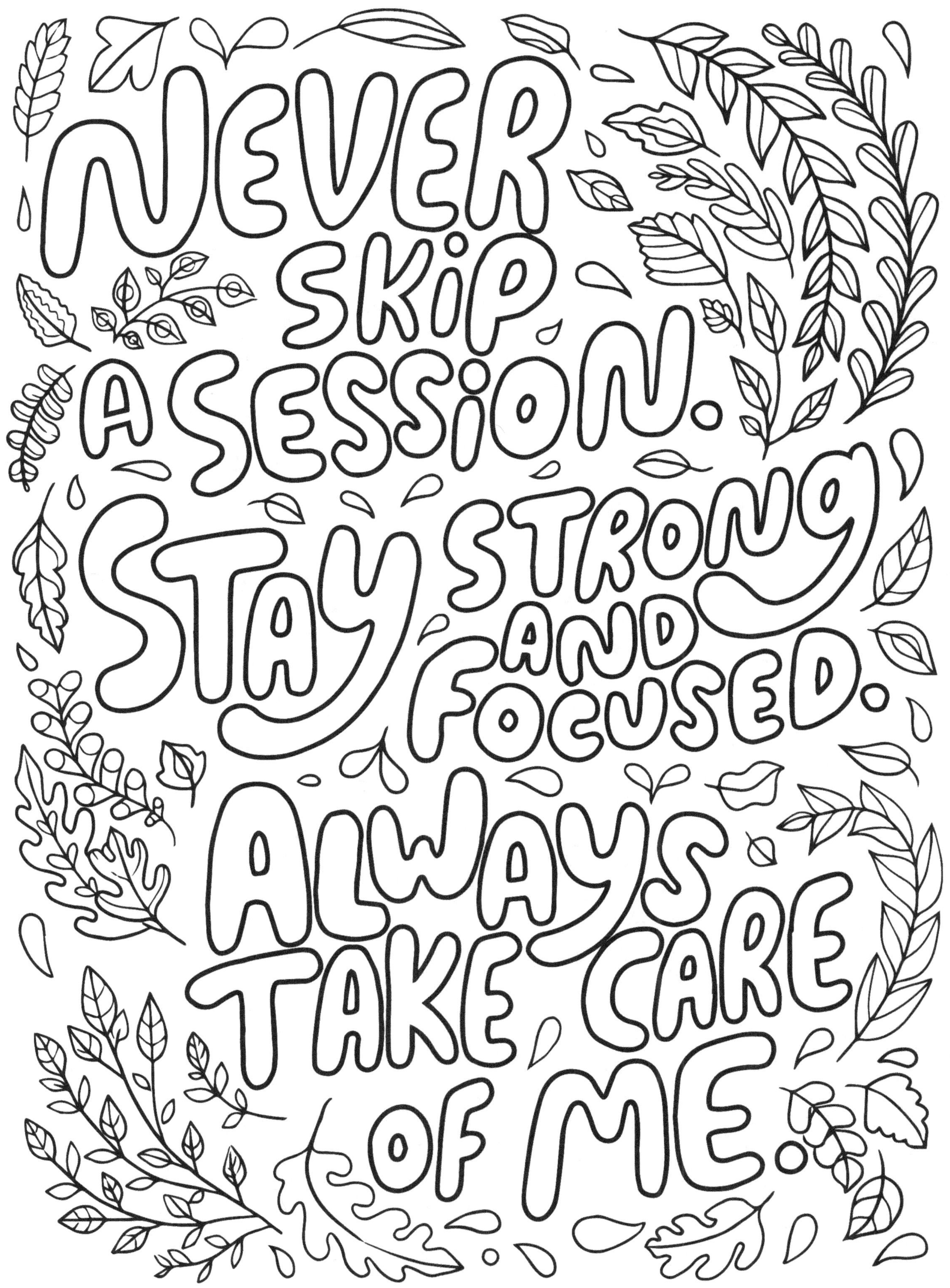

Never skip a session.
Stay strong, and focused.
Always take care of me.

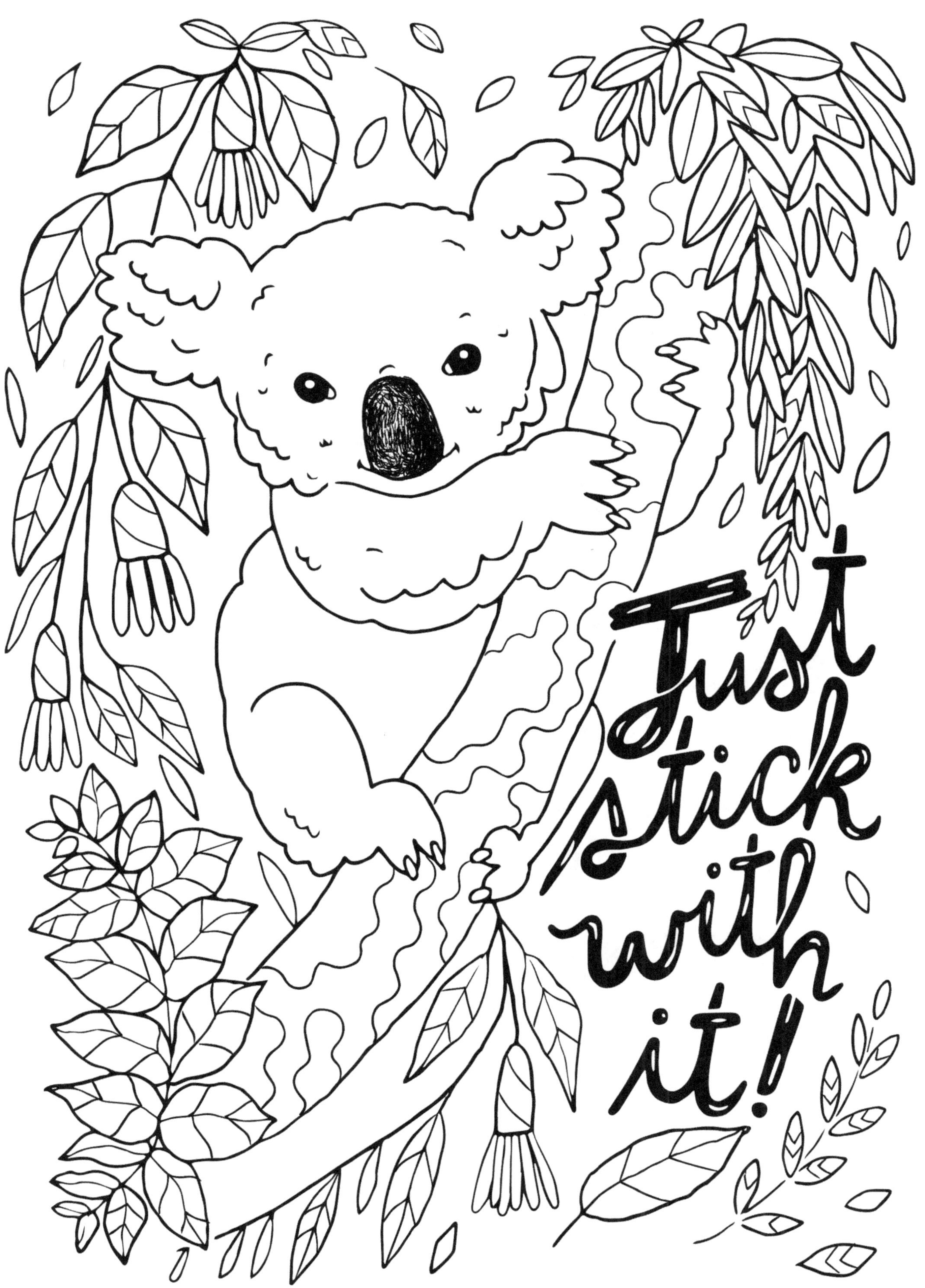
Just
stick
with
it!

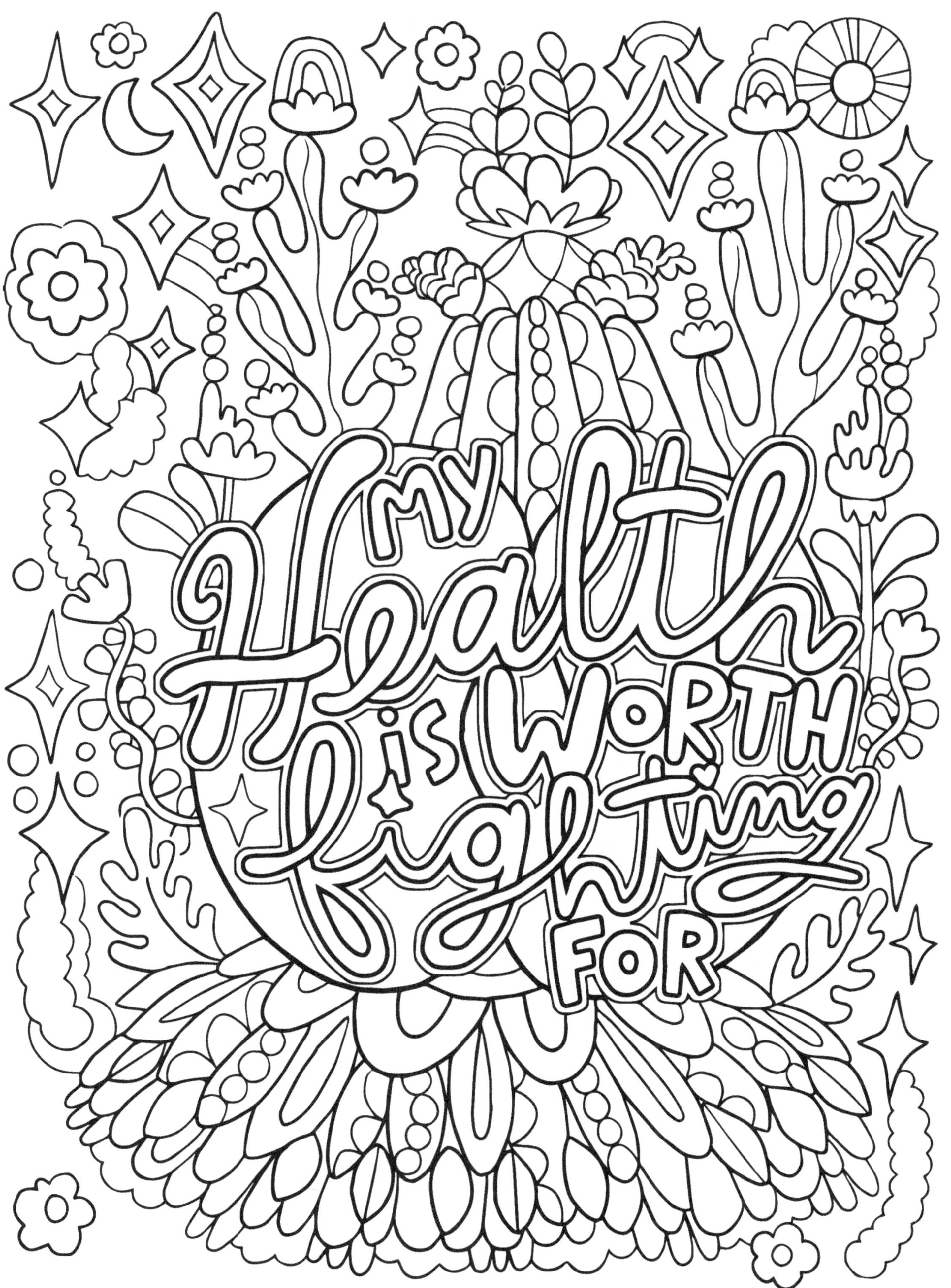

My Health is Worth fighting For

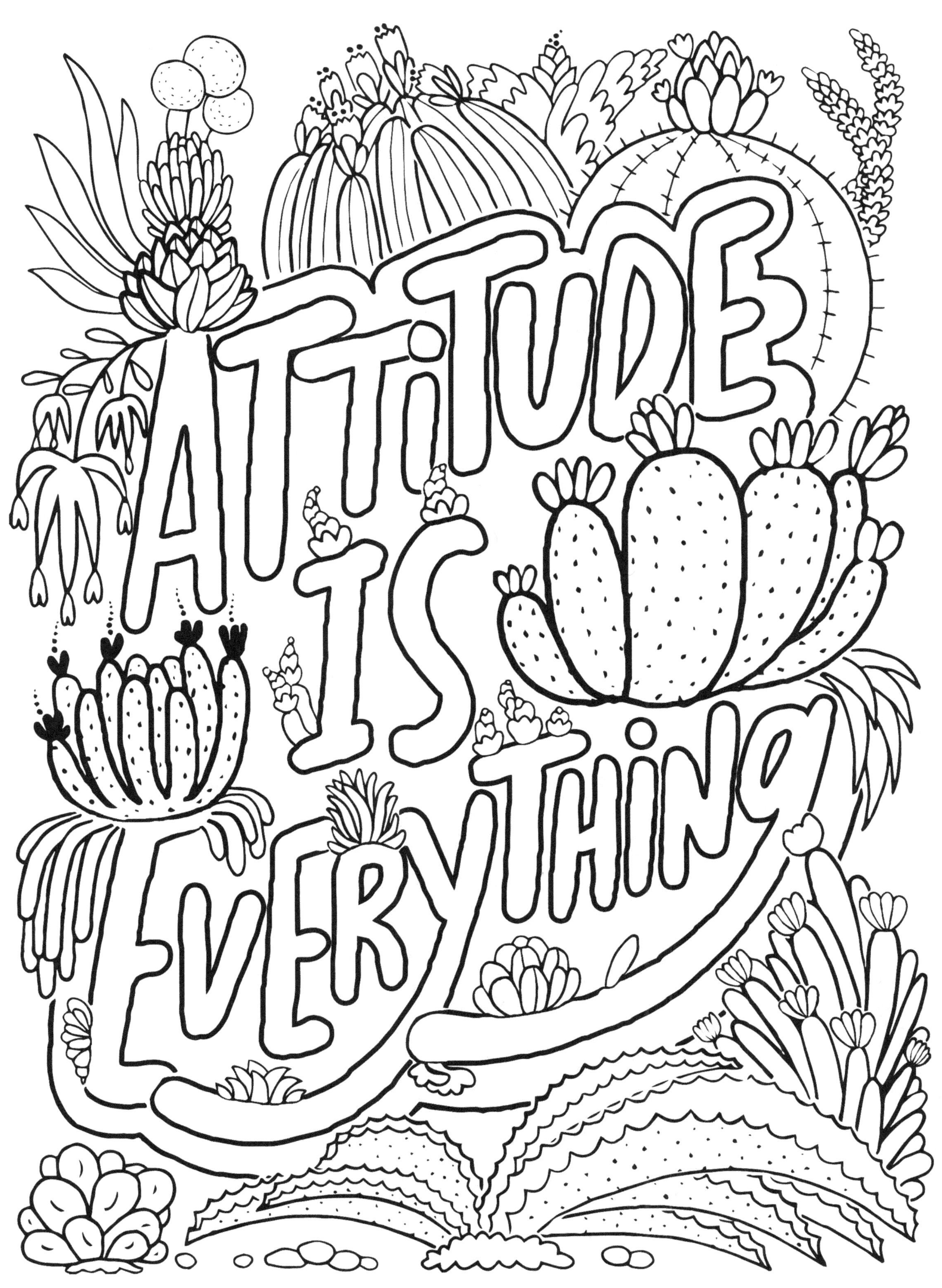

ATTITUDE IS EVERYTHING

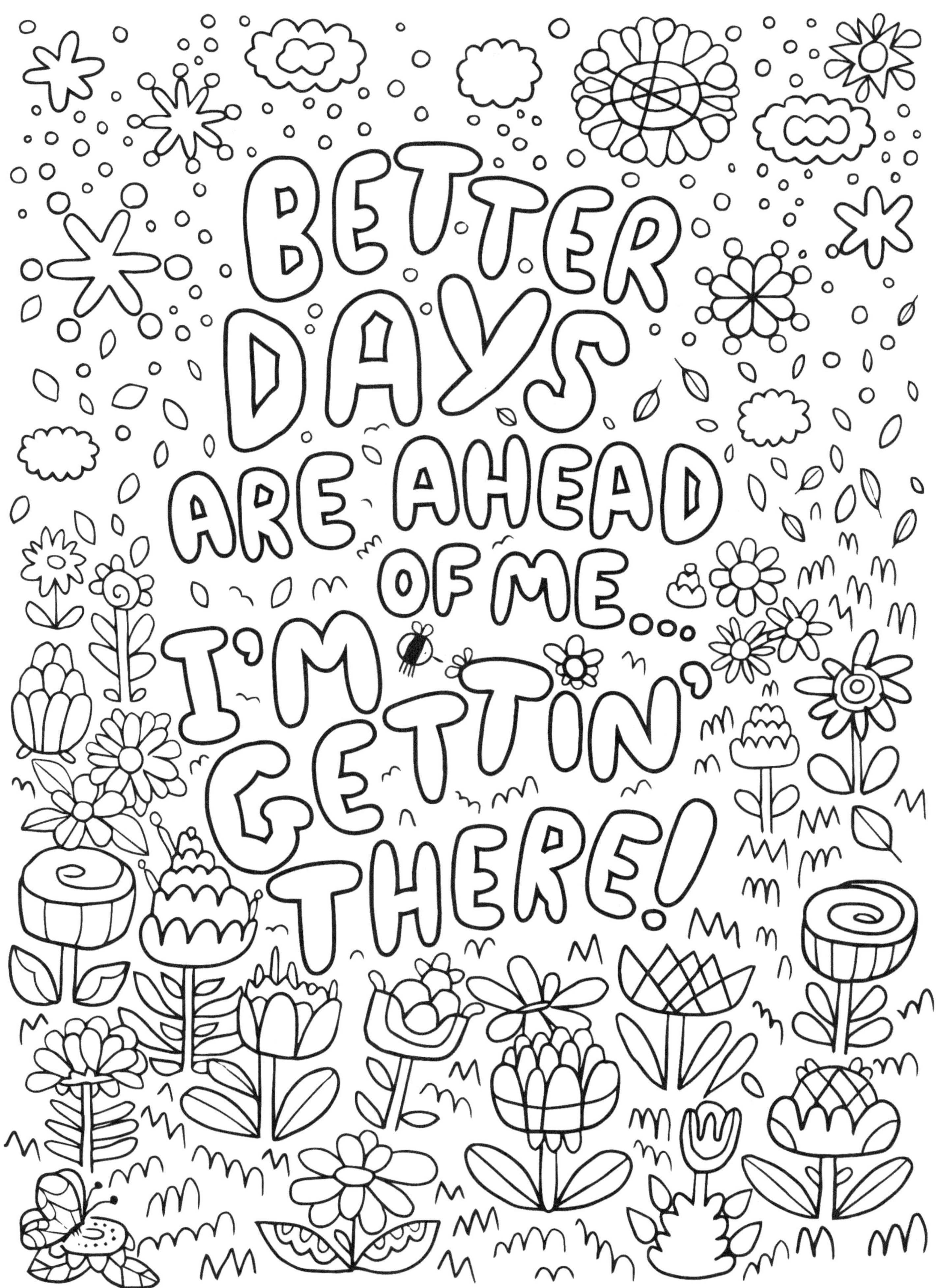

BETTER
DAYS
ARE AHEAD
OF ME...
I'M
GETTIN'
THERE!

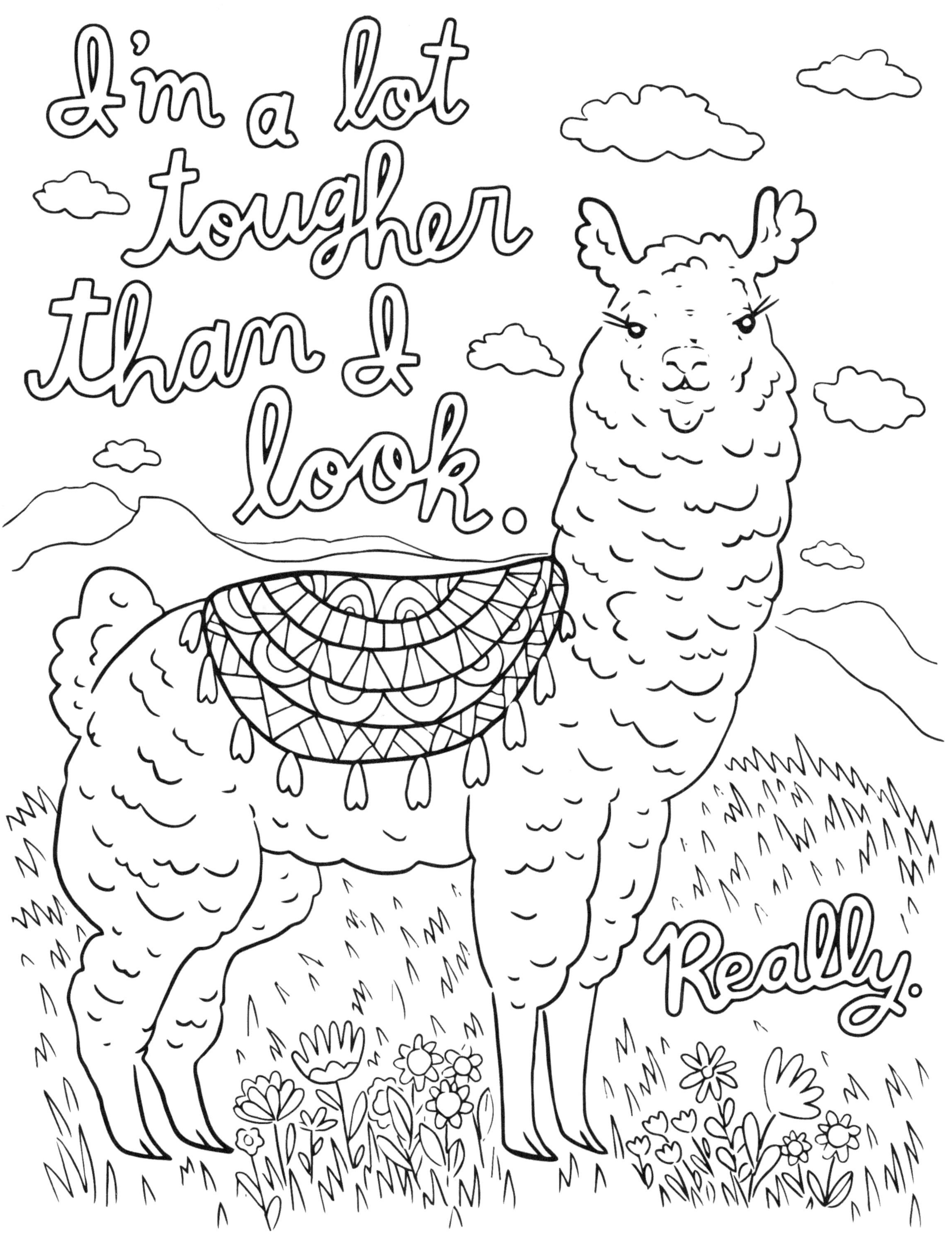

I'm a lot tougher than I look.
Really.

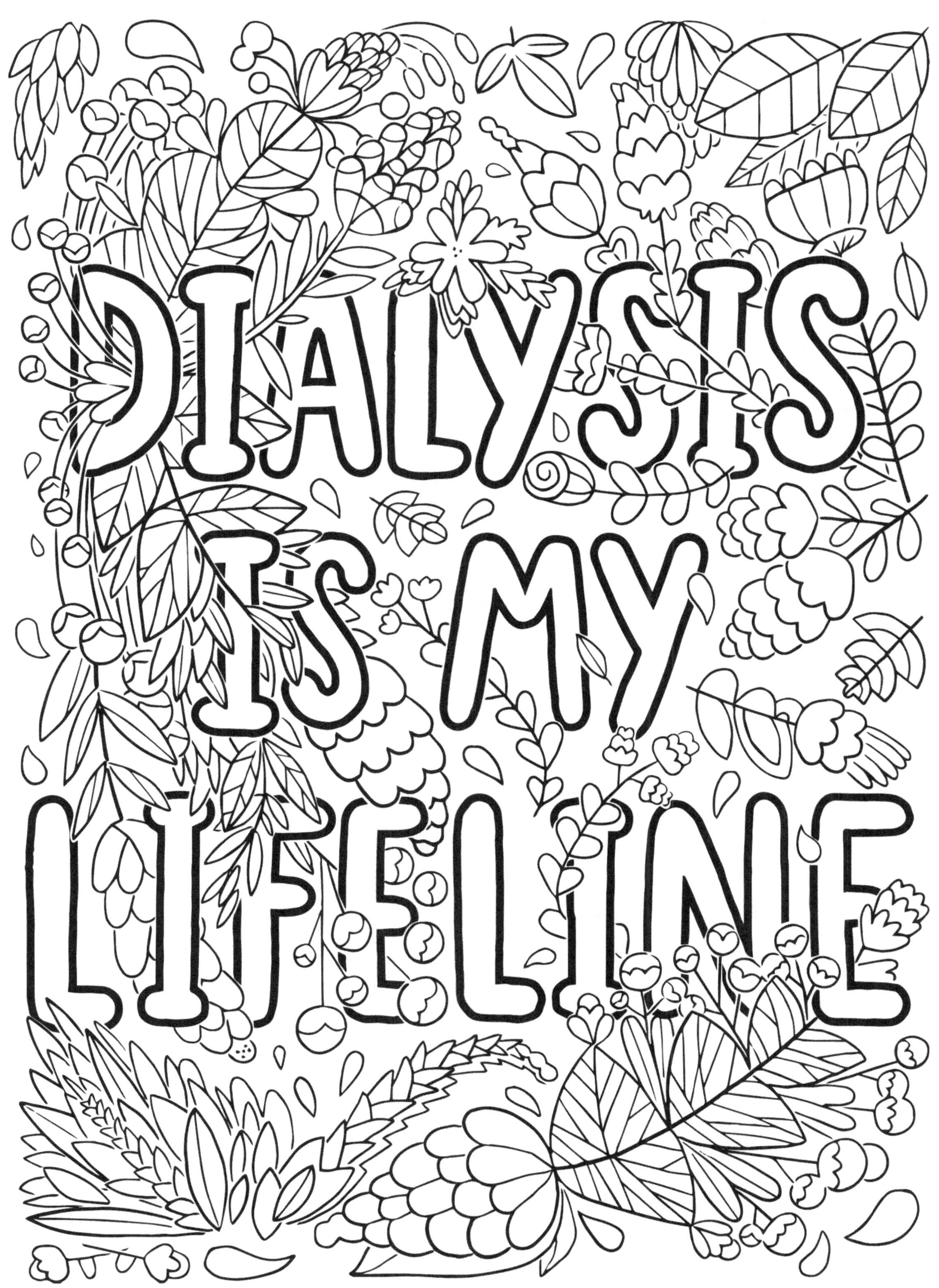

DIALYSIS
IS MY
LIFELINE

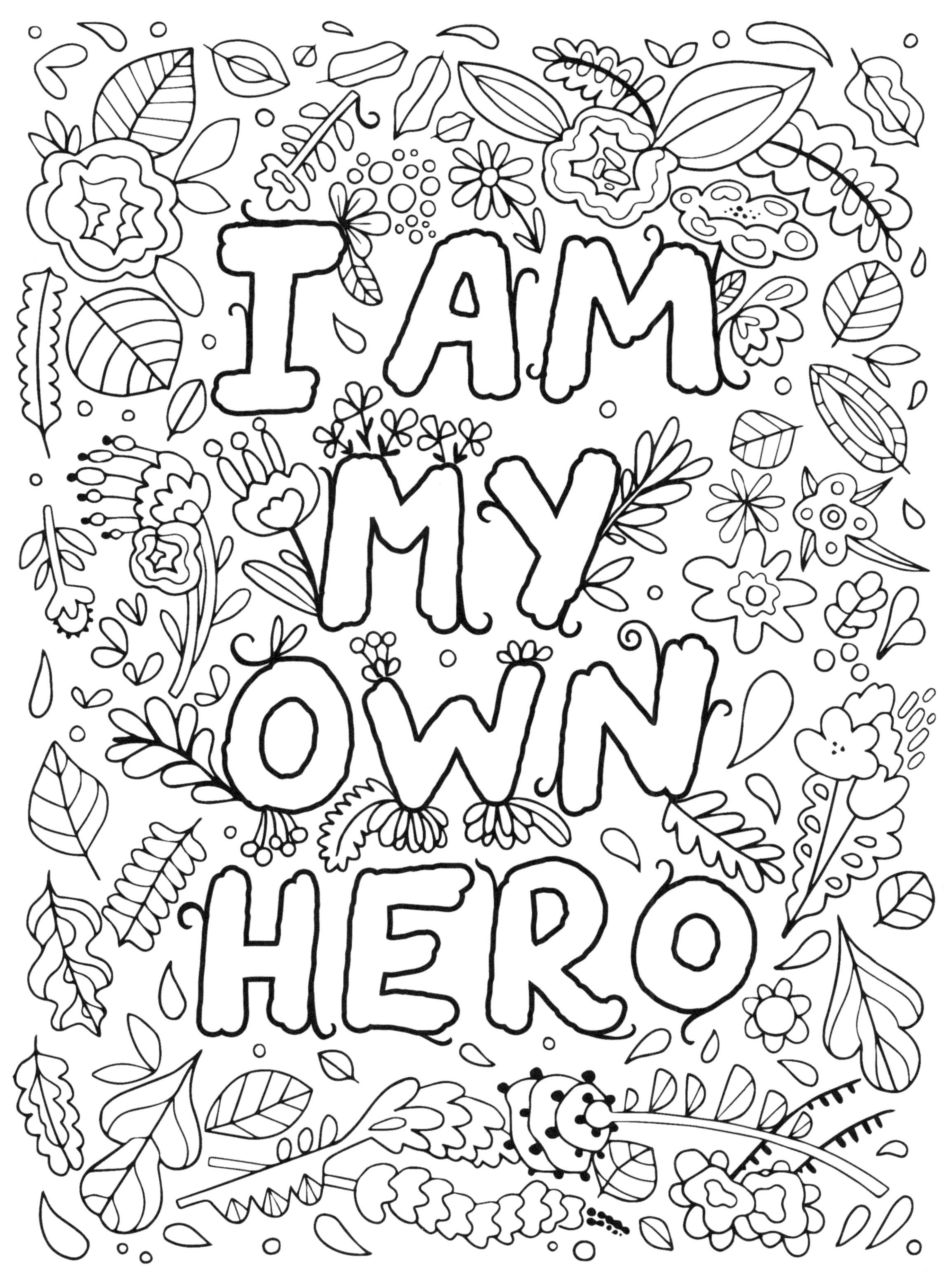

I AM
MY
OWN
HERO

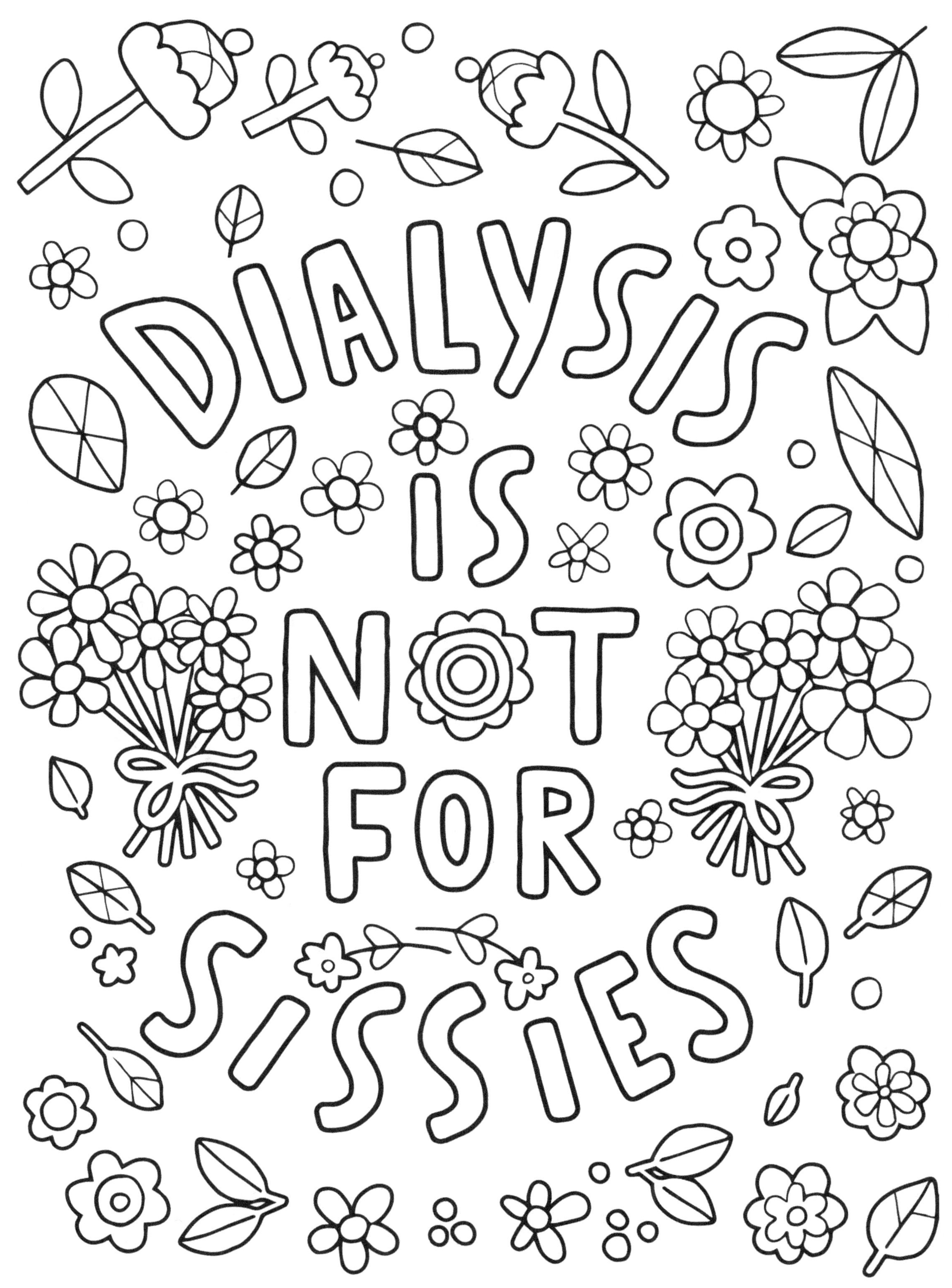

DIALYSIS
IS
NOT
FOR
SISSIES

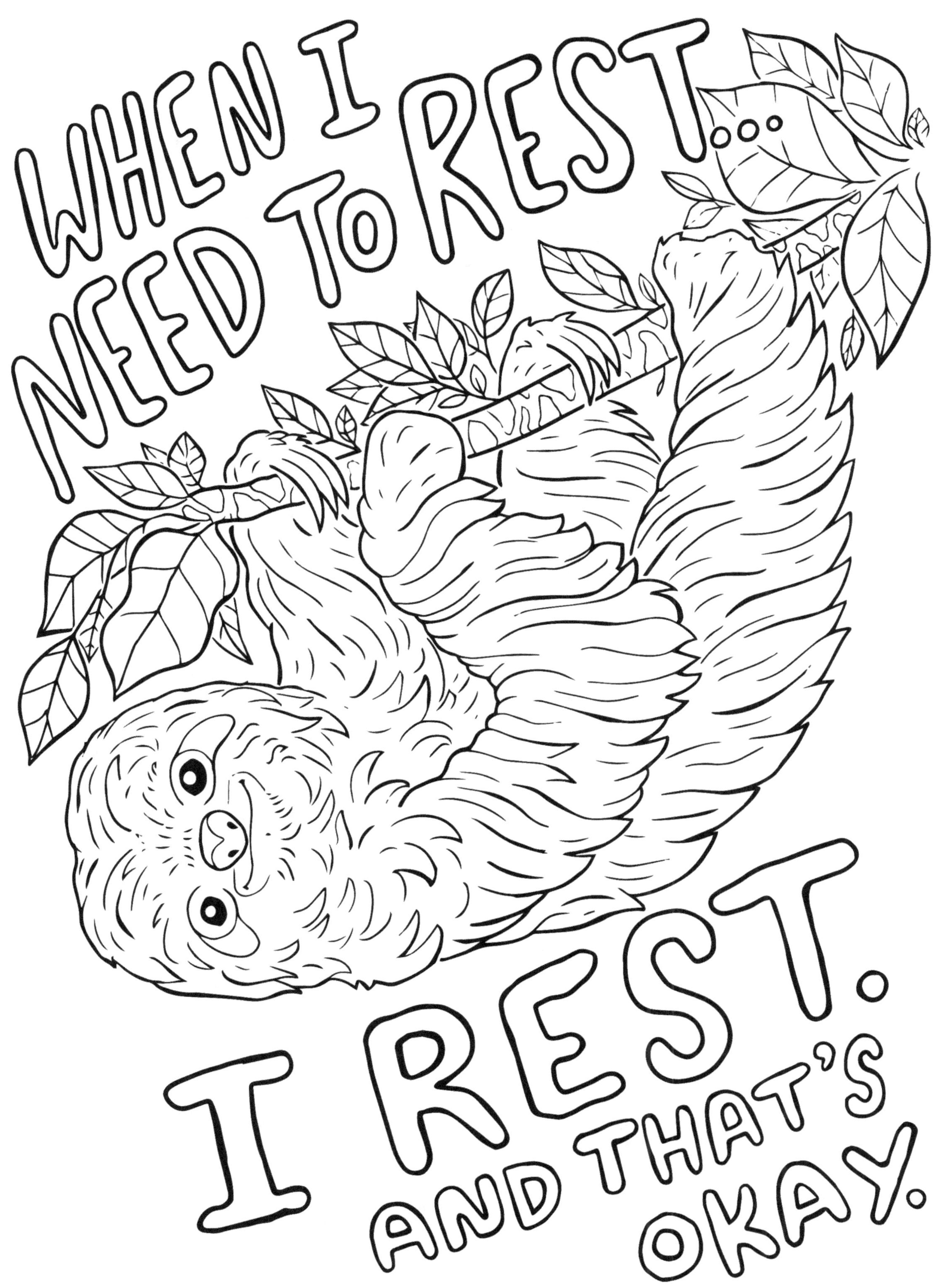

WHEN I NEED TO REST...
I REST.
AND THAT'S OKAY.

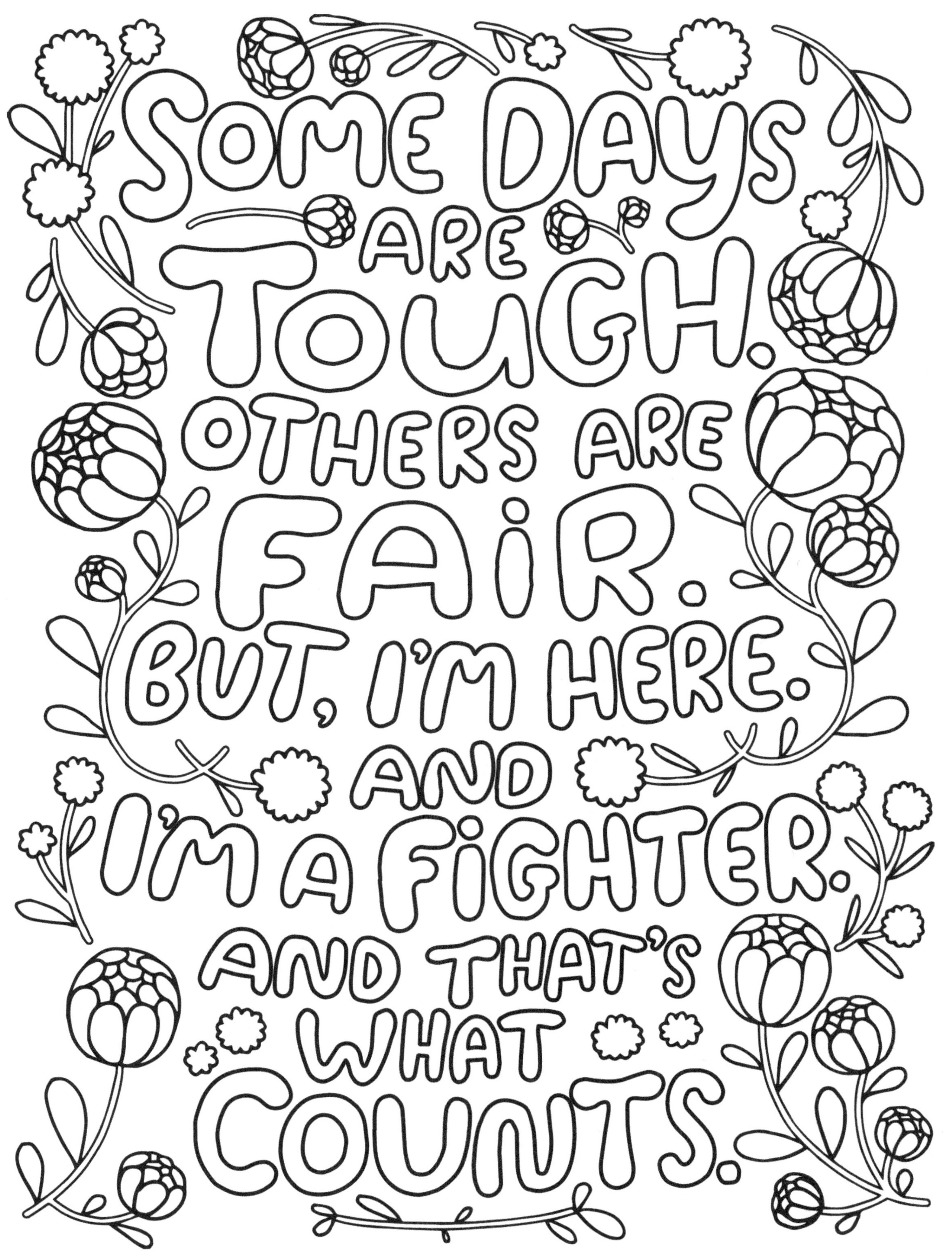

Some Days
are Tough.
Others are
Fair.
But, I'm here.
and
I'm a fighter.
and that's
what
counts.

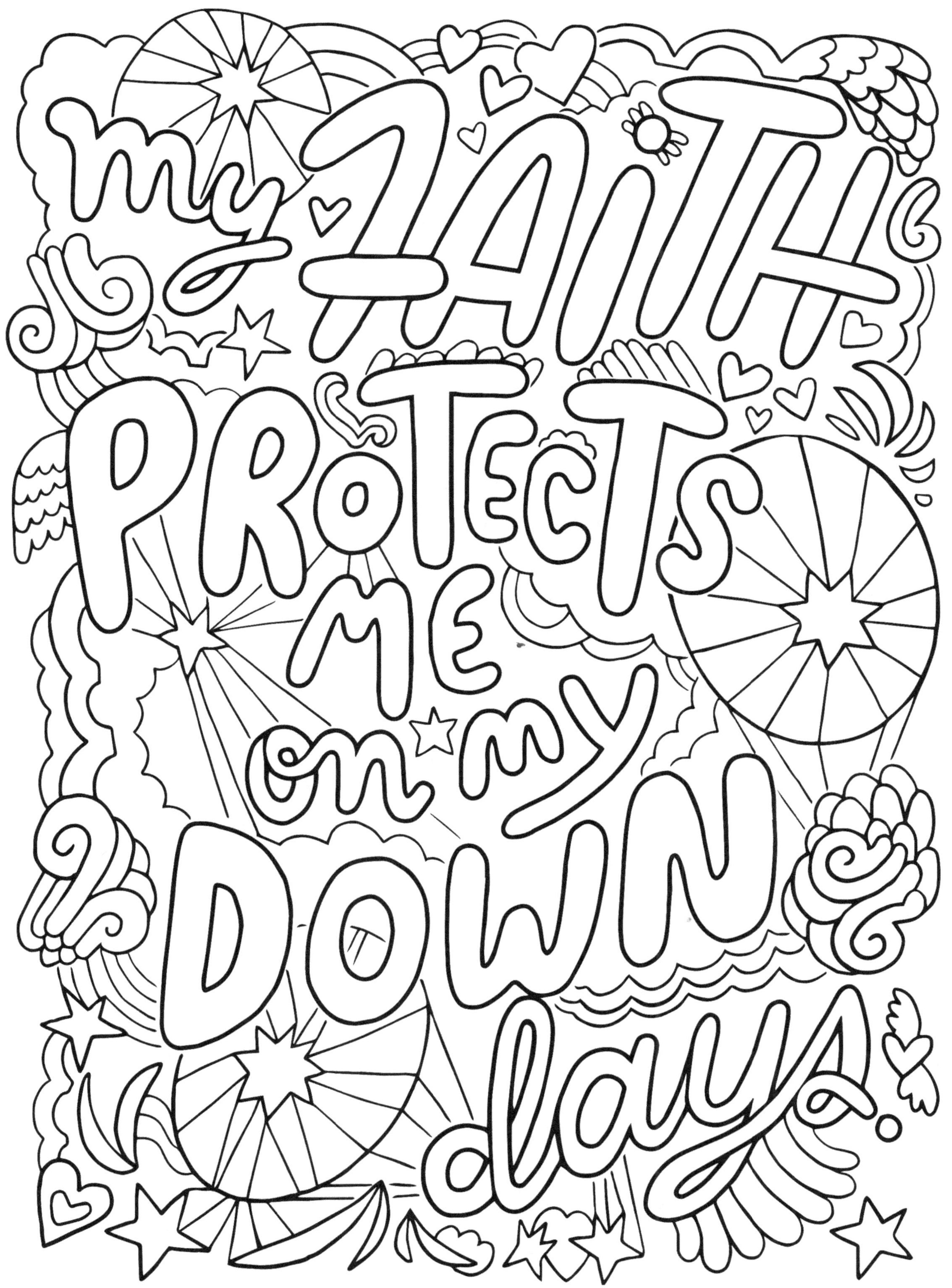

My FAITH
PROTECTS ME
on my
DOWN days

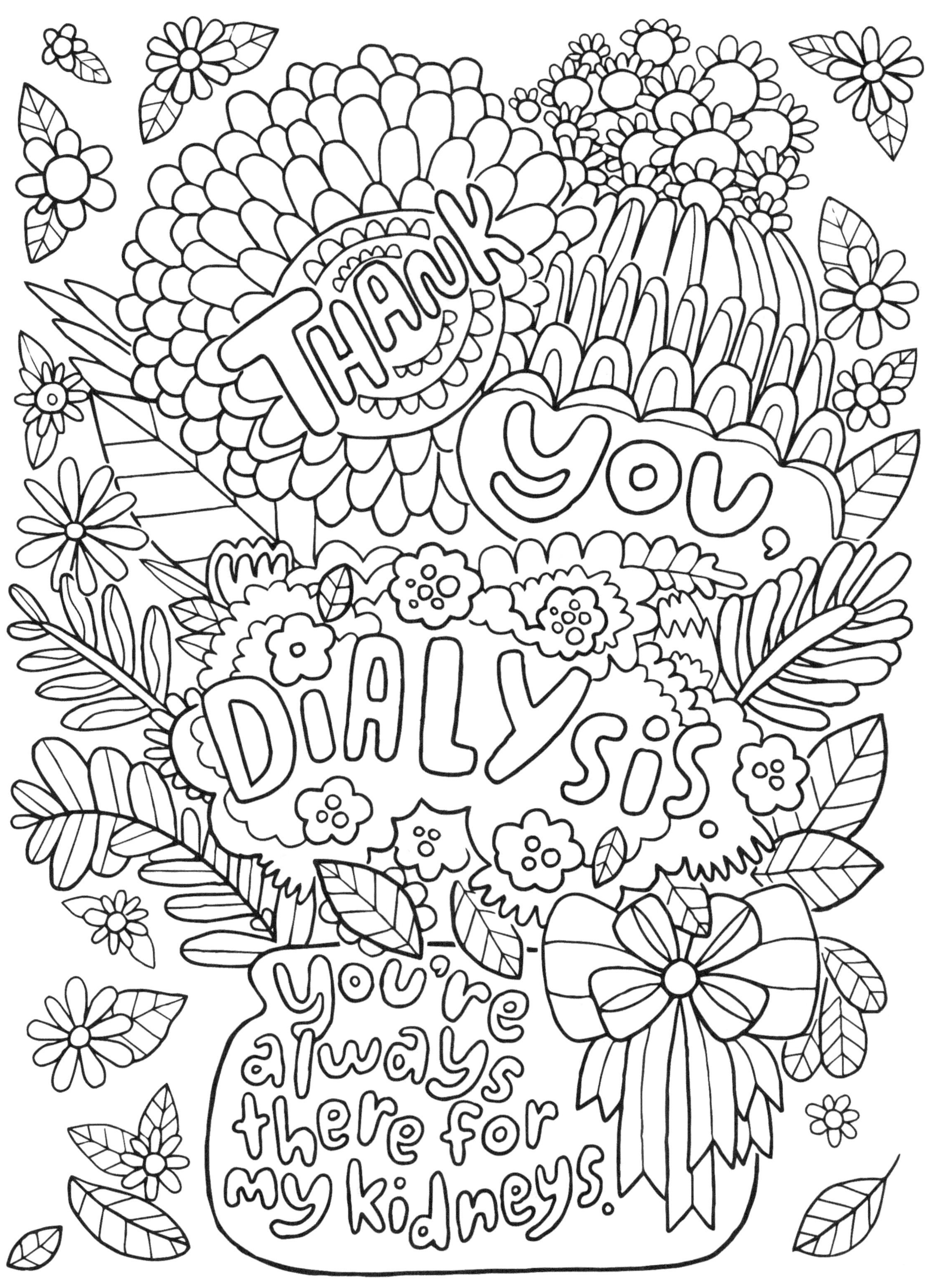
Thank
you,
Dialysis.
You're always there for my kidneys.

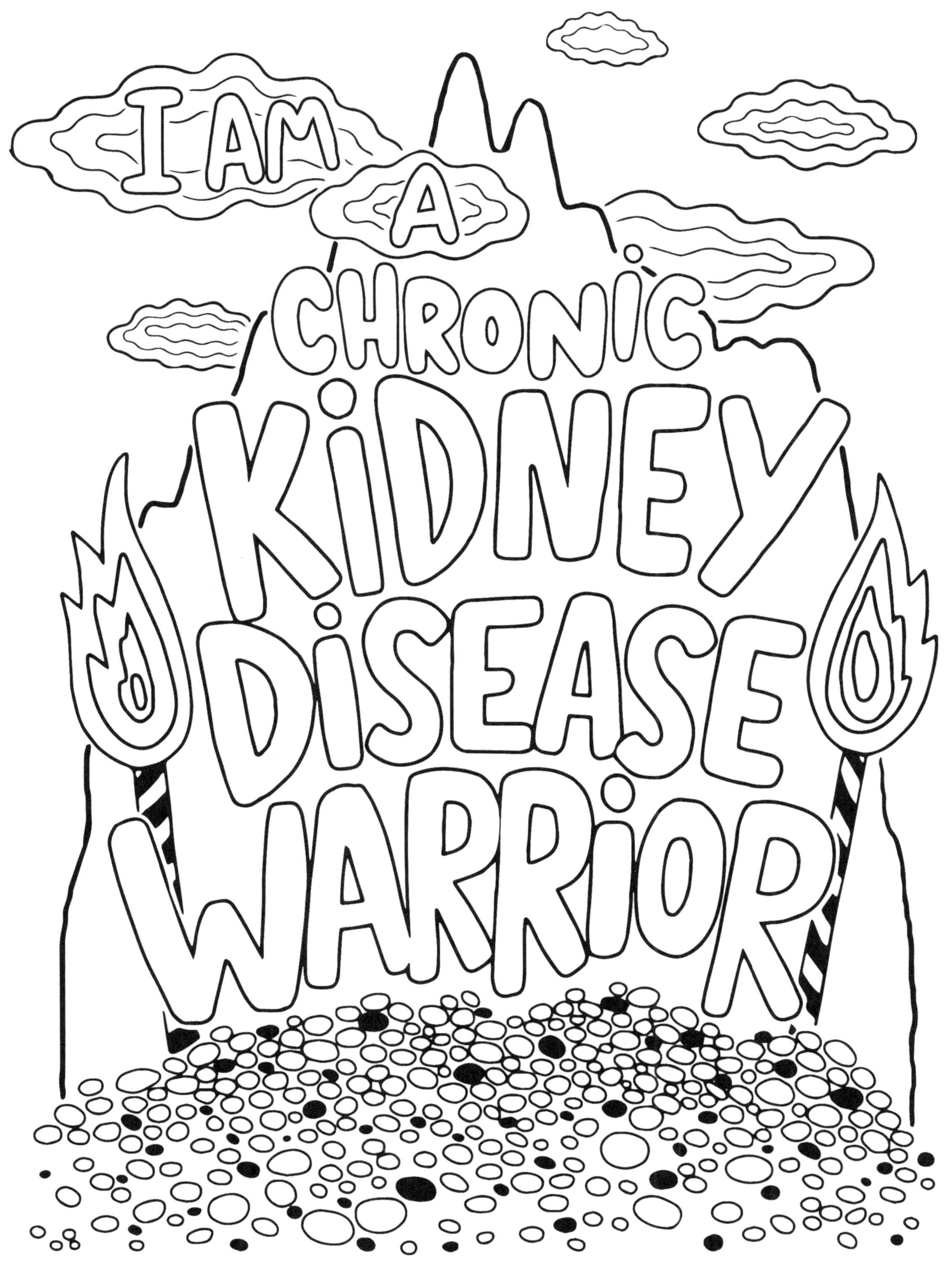

I AM A CHRONIC KIDNEY DISEASE WARRIOR

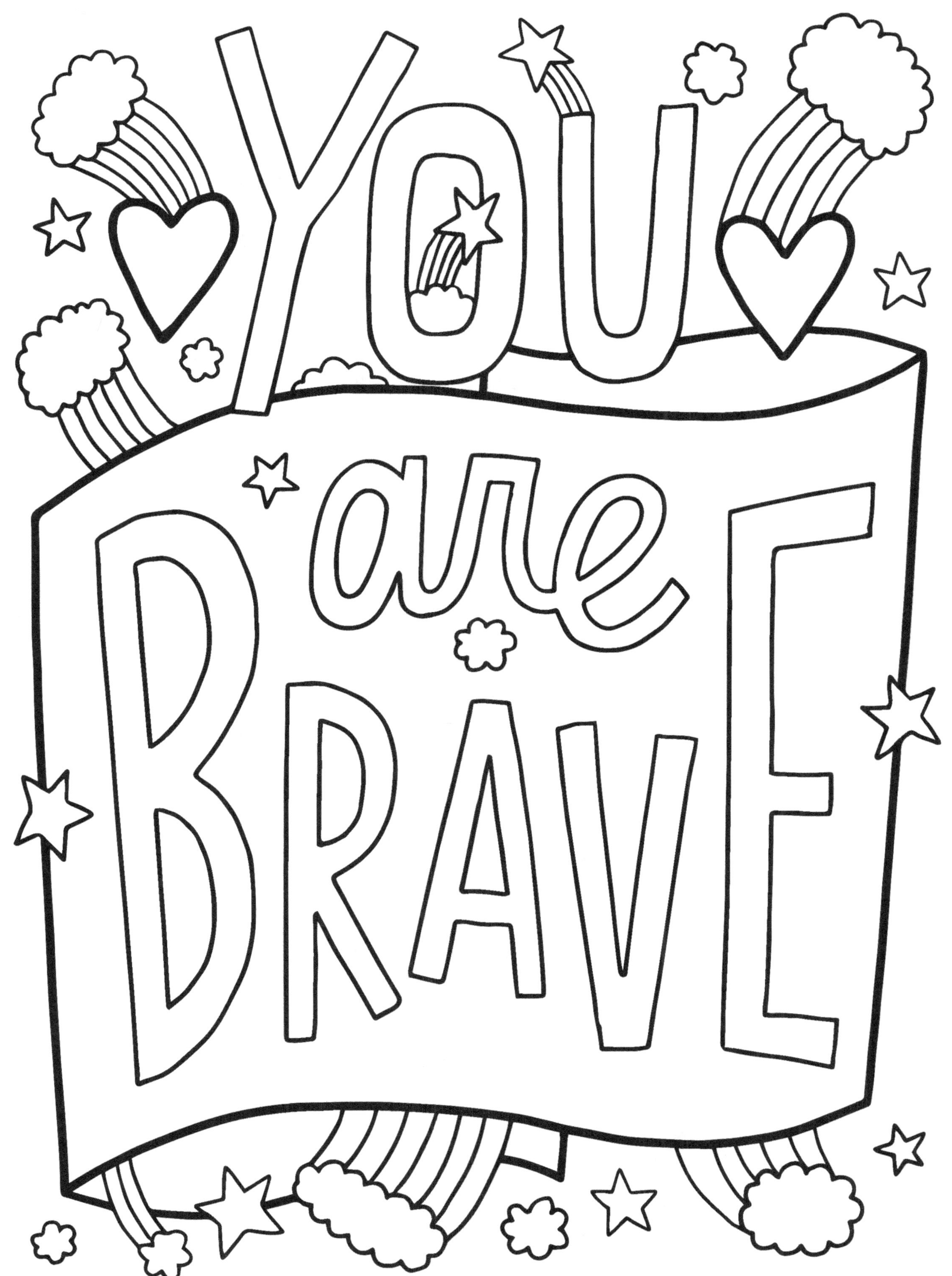

You
are
BRAVE

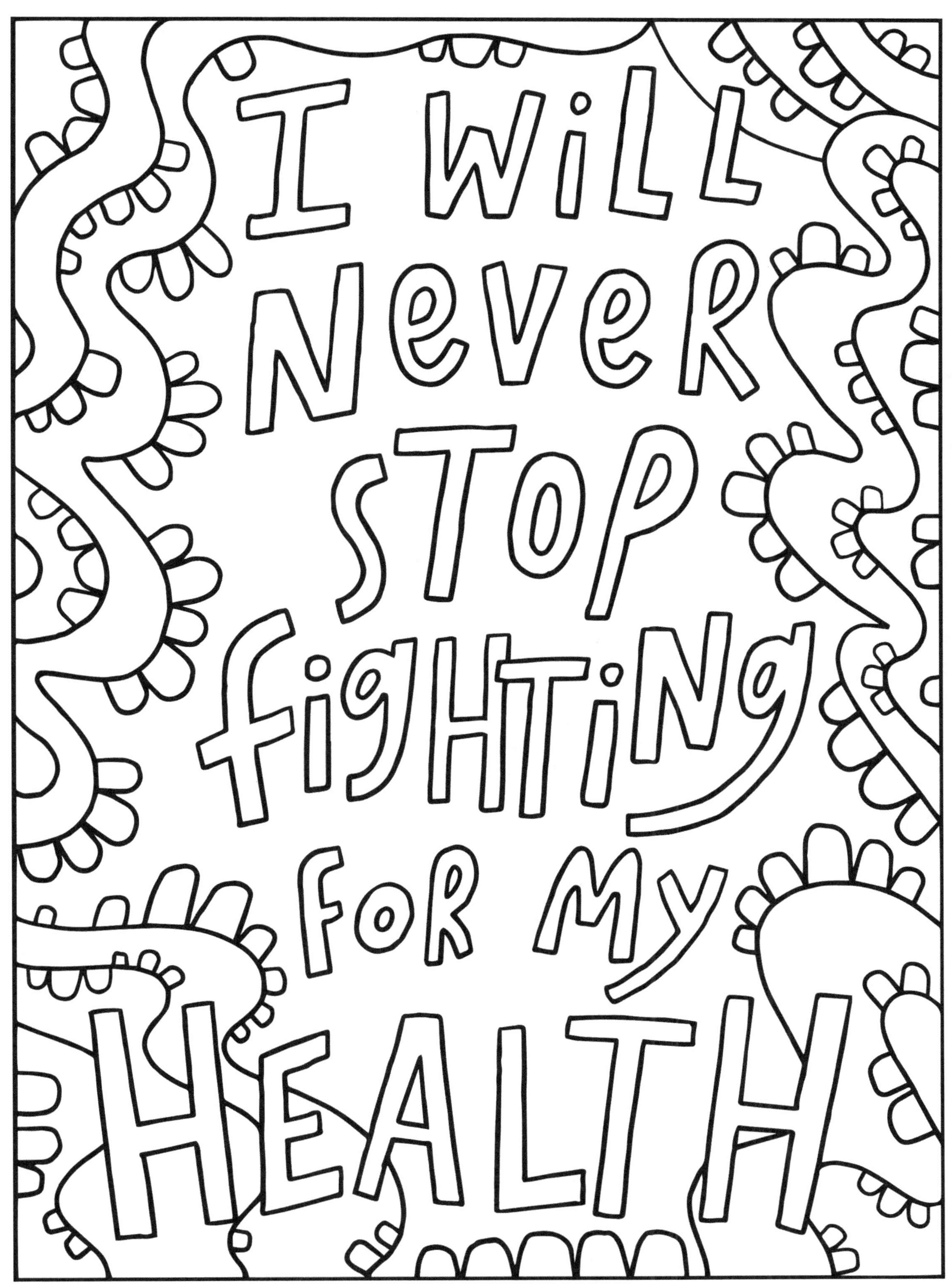

I WILL NEVER STOP FIGHTING FOR MY HEALTH

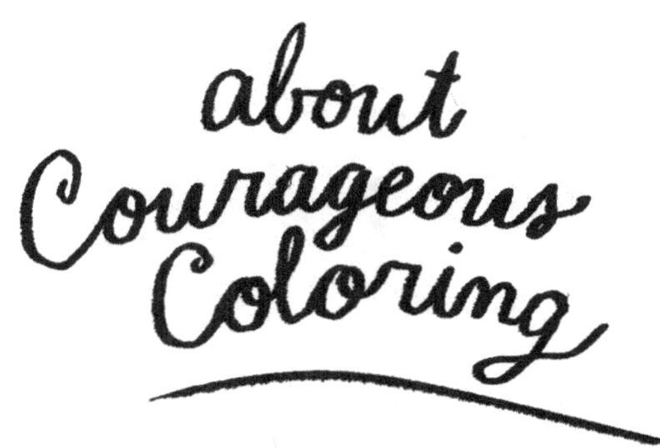

I started Couageous Coloring to encourage creative exploration and discovery for everyone, without self-criticism or judgement.
Get encouraged, motivated, and inspired with Courageous Coloring!

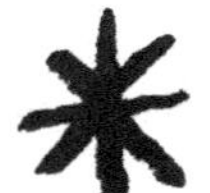 **I Am A Kidney Disease Warrior** is the third coloring book in this series.

Also available:

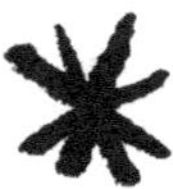 I Am A Cancer Warrior

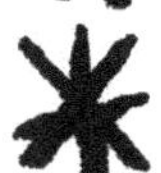 I Am A Chronic Illness Crusader

For more releases, please visit

CourageousColoring.com

If you are enjoying this book...

Please leave an Amazon review. People just like you are shopping Amazon right now, looking for a coloring book just like this one. The more reviews this book has, the more visible Amazon will make it to others shopping for similar books. Reviews that include photos or videos of your beautiful coloring pages are extremely appreciated!!

let's connect!

Coloring books 

courageouscoloring.com
shop.kathyweller.com
kathywellerart.etsy.com

facebook 

facebook.com/**kathywellerart**

Twitter

twitter.com/**kathywellerart**
twitter.com/**courageouscolor**

Instagram 

instagram.com/**kathywellerart**
instagram.com/**courageouscoloring**
instagram.com/**shopkathyweller**

main site 

kathyweller.com

art videos

youtube.com/**kathywellerart**